The New Nurse Handbook:

Navigating Your First Year as a Nurse

- By Jay Nichols (BSN, RN, DNP-S)

Table of Contents

About the Author

Jay Nichols, known on social media as Jay Quinn is a Critical Care Nurse in the US Air Force. She is a graduate of the University of South Carolina Mary Black School. She started her nursing career as a new graduate when she moved from South Carolina to Rochester, MN for a new grad nursing position in the Medical/Surgical ICU unit at the Mayo Clinic.

In January 2018, Jay began her journey once again as a student in an accredited Acute Care Nurse Practitioner Doctoral Program. Jay seeks to mentor nurses and nursing students alike, helping them reach their fullest potential. With the use of social media, Jay uses her platform to help encourage, engage, and spread diversity within the nursing culture. Jay loves spending time with her family traveling, being active, and has a strong relationship with God.

Apart from this book, Jay is the author of the following online publications:

- 10 Benefits of Joining Professional Nursing Organizations and Associations

- 3 Tips on How to be a Critical Care Nurse for New Grad Nurses
- My NCLEX Experience: Study Tips and Resources for Nursing Students

You can connect with Jay on the following platforms:

Website: www.ontargetnurse.com

Instagram:@jvogue92

YouTube: www.youtube.com/jayquinn92

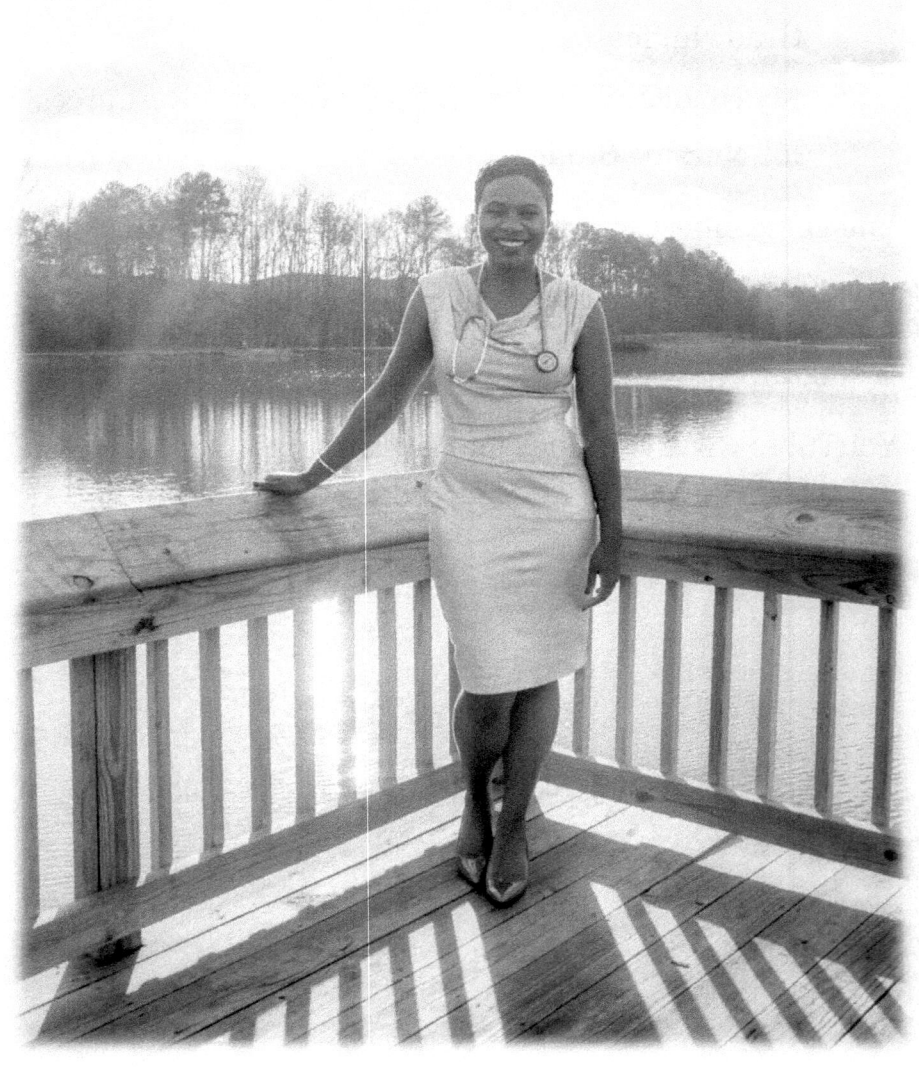

Acknowledgements

I want to thank God first and foremost for this opportunity and for allowing me to continue to reach new heights every day.

I want to thank my parents; Jerry & Maria, and my brother Quincey for their constant love, support and encouragement.

I want to thank Nurses in my life who I know personally and those I have encountered as a student, and during my professional career who have shown endless support, encouragement, and professionalism. It's your mentoring and love for the profession that have encouraged me.

I want to thank everyone who is reading this, thank you for taking the time to support me as well as yourself! You are all an inspiration to me!

Introduction

Congratulations on taking the first steps in your new career as nurse. Nursing is a very rewarding profession that has drastically changed over the last few decades. In spite of all the changes within the nursing profession, it still offers rich and diverse opportunities. After my year as a new graduate nurse I felt inspired and encouraged to continue on in my career as a nurse. Unfortunately, that isn't the case for everyone. I'm inspired to encourage and uplift you and the future of nursing as you enter this great profession. I have never for a minute regretted becoming a nurse. Your journey will be paved with moments of great joy and even immense sorrow. You will develop a deep appreciation for life and a respect for death. This guide will help you be well prepared for securing that new job you have been searching for as well as provide you with guidance during your first year as a new nurse! I personally want to welcome you in into the nursing profession, wish you immense success as you follow and pursue your dreams.

Any new graduate will have a tough transition from classroom to work place. That is doubly true for nurses, who have to grow up in a career where life and death issues are the norm, not the exception. According to author Barbara Arnoldussen, RN, MBA, the pathway to a successful nursing career starts long before your first day on the job. To insure that you get started on the right foot in your new career newly minted nurses need to be deliberate and prepared at every step along the path to landing that first job.

Unless we are making progress in our nursing

Every year, every month, every week,

Take my word for it,

We are going back

-Florence Nighingale (May 1872)

Landing Your First Job

So, you've passed your NCLEX and now it's time to enter the nursing profession. Getting started might be a bit overwhelming at first since there are so many career avenues to explore. Once you have an idea of the type of position you want and where you want to work, you can start looking for specific positions. Check the qualifications to see what is required for the job you are applying for. For instance, it might be physically demanding, which could pose a challenge for you. Or, some jobs might want candidates that have prior experience.

Today, more than ever, an abundance of opportunities exist for new graduate registered nurses (RNs) in large health systems across the country. However, the new graduate nurse recruitment and hiring market remains competitive.

The first year of your nursing profession can be nerve-wracking and exciting. There are so much new possibilities to discover as you journey the path of being a BSN nurse.

Of course, you know that you want to work as a nurse, but there are a number of different types of nursing jobs out there. Is it your preference to work in a hospital setting? Would you prefer caring for the elderly in a nursing home? Did you hear about an open position with a local health care facility? Perhaps your dream job is to be a school nurse? Do you yearn for the adventure that comes with being a travel nurse?

These are just a few of the questions to ask yourself as you begin your job search. If you're open to all of the above, you'll have more options from which to choose, of course. Here are some places where employment opportunities may be available:

- Area hospitals
- Clinics
- Nursing homes, residential care providers, or rehabilitation centers

- Health insurance providers
- Travel nursing agencies
- Home health care agencies
- Local government agencies

Once you have an idea of the type of position you want and where you want to work, you can start looking for specific positions. Many career experts advise new nurses to conduct targeted job searches through job boards specific to your area of expertise.

You should develop a plan that includes a great deal of exploration and investigation. Colleges and universities do a great job of providing nursing students with on-site recruitment events. Healthcare organizations often travel near and far to attend these events and meet with soon-to-be new graduates (as well as undergraduates). Although these opportunities provide a one-stop shop, they can be overwhelming, thus having an interview plan is essential.

I think breaking the plan into two parts will be a great idea: Plan A and Plan B. If a new graduate has a strong desire to work at a certain hospital in a certain unit (Plan A), such as where they spent clinical time for example, and that opportunity does not exist, the new graduate should have an alternate plan in place (Plan B). Plan B should be a position that will provide the experience needed to help develop the skills that will allow an eventual move to Plan A. One of the many great things about the profession of nursing is that each and every position and experience creates another layer of expertise, skill and knowledge.

Review hospital websites is a very important activity you need to actively engage in in a bid to land that first job. After reviewing a posting, which includes job location, department, status and shift, if you are interested as a new grad, you can □uickly and easily complete the application in its entirety. Additionally, always have an updated resume and a list of references with contact information on hand when applying for positions.

Thoroughly researching the hospital or healthcare organization is a must. This research can help new graduate RNs formulate questions that can be used during an interview. It is imperative that new graduate RNs are prepared to ask questions when being interviewed. Often, taking the time to prepare carefully thought-out questions, as opposed to generic off-the-cuff questions, can be a huge differentiator when comparing candidates.

Of course, you've probably heard that conventional wisdom that says most people don't get hired after applying to a job posting. In other words, you don't want to really solely on that method. One great source of job leads may come from your own network of friends and family. You might also tap into your former nursing school connections and alumni office to inquire about career leads. The point is that you should actively put yourself out there. You might just strike up a conversation with a neighbor and find out that his sister is a long-time nurse who would be willing to share advice with you.

Additionally, professionalism is key. This includes everything from appropriate attire and punctuality to attentiveness, eye contact and sending a handwritten or emailed thank you note following an interview.

I will discuss more on interview tips that will prove very helpful as you hope to land your very first nursing job.

Interview Tips

You've worked so hard in nursing school and on your exams, and now here you finally are, ready to embark on your nursing career. Interviews are nerve wracking in any situation, but particularly early on your career for a job that really excites you.

For job applicants, the job interview is always the dreadful part of the hiring process. Whether you are hoping to get your first nursing job or already have years of experience but wish to apply for a new job or higher position, you will have to go through a job interview and need to impress your potential employer enough that they will hire you.

Know Where to Go

There's nothing like driving to a job interview and realizing you don't know the exact building where the meeting is being held, or you don't have enough money for the parking meter. If at all possible, map out the fastest route to the interview site and drive there a day or two before your big day; make notes about where to park, whether you'll need change for a parking meter, and be sure to ascertain the exact building where you need to be. If possible, check out the inside of the building and learn the very exact location of the office or room you'll need to report to.

Get Some Sleep

Tomorrow is the interview you have been waiting for. You have the perfect thing to wear, you've prepared for a myriad of interview questions, and you've brushed up on how to overcome any bad habits that might deter your interviewer from offering you the job of a lifetime.

Still, there is one more thing of vital importance you need to do before your interview in the morning, which is getting a good night's sleep.

Sleep is vital to our overall well-being so it shouldn't come as much of a surprise that being well rested before you interview is especially important.

The benefits one gets when sleeping are unmistakable. Your memory will improve greatly, your concentration will become more precise, and your creativity will be sparked anew. These new found qualities are assets when preparing for a job interview.

Losing hours of sleep due to pre-interview anxiety is no fun, and it'll set you back for the day. Practice the best sleep hygiene you can in the several days leading up to your interview. Avoid alcohol and other things that may decrease the quality or quanity of your sleep pattern.

One of your main goals the day before your interview should be to get at least an eight hour sleep. Setting eight hours as a specific goal will help move it up your priority list and ensure it comes to pass.

Sleep deprivation can adversely affect interview performance. When overtired and anxious, you can become tetchy and irritable, traits that will not endear you to a potential employer.

Learn About Your Employer/Company

Researching employers is one of the best ways to become a stand-out candidate during the hiring process. By putting on your detective hat and investigating potential employers, you'll discover details about the employer that will better prepare you for any interview.

Learn everything you can in advance about the employer you are interviewing with—their facilities, their staff, the management, their policies, etc. Consider your strengths and weaknesses as they pertain to this particular job and be prepared to discuss them intelligently.

First and foremost, you should know what the company looks for in a qualified candidate. This enables you to position yourself as the best candidate for the position.

To discover the skills and experience the employer values, read between the lines of their job postings. You can also find out information on the employer's career page to get an idea of the type of employees their desire. In addition, reach out to current employees who work there and ask them about what their employer values most in the workplace.

Nothing frustrates a hiring manager more than when they sit down to interview someone for a job and he or she has no knowledge about the company.

It's a waste of time for the hiring manager and the interviewee. No matter how impressive your resume looks, if you know nothing about the company it shows that you didn't take the time to go above and beyond to try and set yourself apart from other applicants.

Showing that you took the initiative to learn about a company demonstrates that you are enthusiastic and serious about the job; and that not just any job will do. This speaks volumes to the employer and they will most likely reward you for the effort by allowing your candidacy to move to the next round.

Do as much advance research as possible about the company or organization to which you are applying; if you understand their mission, values, recent awards or special recognition, and other aspects of the organization, you will be able to speak with more confidence when asked questions probing your understanding of your potential new employer.

Practice Interview Questions

A job interview will primarily involve you being asked questions to determine if you fit the job position. Answering with confidence and substance will impress any interviewer. Being caught off-guard and answering clumsily or insubstantially will turn-off any interviewer. Most job interviews are the same and stock questions usually include like "Tell me about yourself." When asked this, don't just ramble random things about you. Be relevant and go straight to the point. If you are a new graduate, structure your answers around nursing school and how well you did, what subjects most interested you and relevant experiences and achievements.

Ask a friend, nurse colleague, or family member to play the role of the interviewer, and practice looking them in the eye and responding to the questions that are hardest for you.

Mock interviews provide candidates with an opportunity to test out their interview skills with someone who isn't evaluating them for an actual job. A mock interview may be offered through career services for students or recent alumni, by a career coach or through a local workforce services office for candidates in the process of transitioning to a new opportunity.

No one is the perfect candidate, so mock interviews help you clarify responses to certain questions and help you work on areas where you may have weaknesses. In a real interview, there's often no feedback about your interviewing abilities, so a mock interview is a perfect opportunity to find out why you may be having some difficulty in landing your dream job.

Dress Professionally

Do small things right. Dress smartly, but not overtly fashionably. You don't need to attend the interview using your nursing scrubs, but you must make it known that you know all the current standards of a Certified Nursing

Assistant (CNA), Licensed Practical Nurses (LPN) or RNs (registered nurses). Each and every detail might matter especially when you're facing tons of competition.

It's often true that first impressions matter a lot, but in healthcare job interviews when you only have a few minutes to secure a job, every impression matters. The way you dress for your interview will make a first and lasting impression. It communicates two big things to the interviewer: How you compose yourself professionally, and how seriously you take the work. Remember that you're no longer a student; you're entering a career field where lives may depend on you. Dressing like a professional will convey the message that you understand and are ready for this responsibility.

You certainly want to look good for your interview. Choose clothes that fit well, feel good against your skin, and help you to feel confident, professional, and attractive. You always want to dress as nicely as possible without being over the top formal.

Just like any other job interview the important thing that you need to keep in mind is that you would want the interview to give an impression that you are qualified for the job and that you are the best candidate for the said job. If this is your first job interview it is only normal to feel nervous. Other people might even feel a great anxiety and wouldn't be able to sleep the whole night before the interview. Now, you should keep in mind that you need to be physically and mental ready for the bid day. That is why it is very important to sleep well the night before the job interview. The greatest tool that you can have in an interview is nothing more than to be prepared for anything. If you are prepared for the interview you can be assured that you will be more confident with the stuff that you are talking about and how you showcase your talent.

Your resume should tout your credentials, license, skills, and relevant work experience, whereas your cover letter allows you to go a bit more in-depth as to why you're a good candidate for the position.

The key to standing out from among your fellow applicants is to customize your resume and cover letter for the specific positions to which you're applying. In other words, scan the job qualifications and tweak your master resume and letter so that you make a connection between the employer's needs and what you can offer. You'd be surprised at how few people do this, and therefore end up sending an application that isn't relevant.

*For more information and help on how to create an amazing CV, visit my YouTube channel and view the following video: **Nursing Resume| New Grad or Grad School + Template**

Everything You Need to do Before Your First Day

So, you have got that long awaited call and you have been offered the job! Congratulations! Hopefully, this is the beginning of what is to be a long successful career in nursing.

A nurse plays a crucial role in improving the public's health and well-being. They always put the needs of their patients first and are a critical link between those being treated and the wider medical team. As a nurse, you will have the opportunity to work at different levels of practice, such as a staff nurse or advanced nurse practitioner, and within different specialisms, as a mental health or paediatric nurse for example. Your job will range from purely clinical care to wider emotional and social support and can take you into education, training and management.

Every role has its unique job description, you should read and re-read your own roles and responsibilities. It is very important that you are fully aware of your duties so you can perform them diligently within your specific position.

Understand the Nurse Practice Act

The Nurse Practice Act is essentially your nursing rulebook! Each state has its own Nurse Practice Act that you must learn, know and live by when working as a registered nurse in the USA. The Nurse Practice act ensures that all registered nurses are qualified and competent of doing their job to the highest standard.

Each Nurse Practice Act:

- Outlines its definitions
- Outlines the Authority, Power and Composition of the state Board of Nursing (BON)

- Sets out the standards for educational programs
- Sets out the standards and scopes of nursing practice
- Outlines the types of titles and licenses, and the protection of these titles and requirements needed for licensure
- Outlines the grounds for disciplinary action and other violations.

The intimate nature of nursing means that the risk of accidents is high. The laws and regulations set out in a states Nurse Practice Act have been put together to reduce the risk of harm to patients and to protect patients by ensuring the highest level of competence. The Nurse Practice Act aims to ensure that patients are receiving quality care and promotes patient safety.

Obtain Professional Liability Insurance

Professional liability insurance, also called errors and omissions or professional indemnity insurance, protects service businesses from the cost of defending negligence lawsuits and other claims of service-related errors.

Succeeding in a service industry or profession can be difficult. You always strive to do your best work and keep your clients happy. But sometimes, no matter how well you assess a client's situation, things don't go according to plan.

As a practicing nurse, you should consult with an attorney or insurance agent to advice you on how to go about obtaining your professional liability insurance. It will help cover you in case of lawsuits for alleged mistake or failure to act.

Prepare Your Positive Attitude

Read through any contracts, induction packs, or emails you have received. These will have important information about your employment, responsibilities, and what you may need to bring with you when you start. When you are familiar with your job description, you will be able to work more safely and efficiently.

If you've graduated from nursing school, one would assume you're quite teachable at this point. Never let this habit fade. You'll be surrounded by seasoned nurses who have a wealth of knowledge. Absorb the lessons they're willing to share and apply them immediately.

Orientation Process

Most hospitals will offer an orientation/internship program for new grad nurses. During my time as a new grad nurse at the Mayo Clinic, I was not only on orientation with my unit but also included in the new nurse residency program. This is a vital time in your career. A time to learn the ins and outs of your facility. A time to hone in on important clinical skills, gain experience, ask questions, and learn about your new unit all while under the wings of your preceptor.

Most hospital-based nursing orientation programs will include a general orientation in the classroom followed by an orientation on the unit you were hired to work on.

A preceptor or mentor is a registered nurse, preferably with a BSN degree, who has been working at the institution for at least two years. The unit orientation can vary in length of time depending on the health care institution. You generally will be on orientation following your preceptor/mentor's schedule for about three to six months. If you were hired to work in a critical care area, your orientation will most likely be longer and even up to one year depending on the facility.

It is important to remember that the health care facility wants to make your orientation a successful one. A successful orientation program helps ensure your competency caring for patients and improves both nurse recruitment and retention at the facility. You are now ready to begin the interview process, and always keep in mind why you were called to the wonderful world of nursing.

Preceptor Tip – You will either work with one preceptor very closely during the duration of your orientation or have a few preceptors. To get the most out of our orientation, always ask questions about what you don't know! Use the preceptor's feedback to work on areas of improvement. Don't feel pressured into doing anything you haven't been trained on or don't feel comfortable with, and definitely don't take any form of preceptor bullying!

Best Work Habits

No matter, whether you're a new graduate or an experienced nurse, the first day at a new job or new location can be exciting, stressful, or overwhelming.

There is so much to learn in addition to the duties or responsibility related to the job. If you are a new graduate, congratulations on your first job! This is your chance to begin your career in health care.

Look and Listen

Situational awareness will go a long way in your nursing career. Make sure you take plenty of time to observe the unit. Listen to how the team communicates. Watch how the team works together. Adjust how you work and communicate accordingly. Remember, it's your job to adjust to your surroundings – not the other way around.

Show You Are Reliable

A great way to prove you can be trusted is to show up on time. Better yet, show up at least 20 minutes early! Review patient charts ahead of your shift and ask for feedback from your preceptor. Taking the initiative will go a long way towards demonstrating you the right person for the job.

Humor Yourself

In the right context, humor can be an excellent way to ease your patient's (and your) nerves. Find humor wherever you can.

Be a Team Player

This one is needs little explanation. Offer to help before being asked. Lend yourself to your fellow nurses. You'll quickly gain the trust and respect of your coworkers.

Give it Time

It's normal to feel overwhelmed as a new nurse. Nursing school can only prepare you for so much. Take the lumps in stride, adapt, be fluid, and grow. This is the first step in what should be a long and meaningful career, so give yourself time to get acclimated.

Get Yourself Ready

Look for comfortable and durable scrubs that make you look professional. You should also plan to wear comfortable shoes that offer strong arch support and a roomy toe box, in addition to heels that do not pinch or slip and a no-slip sole.

Be Polite

You will encounter the whole array of human emotions on the floor, ranging from sadness to excitement. Be polite to your patients, peers and strangers you meet at the elevators. You never know when one of them could become your next patient. You represent something greater than yourself; you represent the hope of feeling better.

Reward Yourself After You Clock Out

Your first day on the floor will be exciting, tiring and rewarding. You could encounter something your instructors never dreamed of seeing, or you could save someone's life. When it is time to clock out, reward yourself for becoming part of an amazing group of people who spring to action when others feel like giving up.

How to Stay Organized

If you're a nurse, you know there is never enough time to get everything done. While you can't change the number of hours in your day, you can change how you use time to maximize every minute. This doesn't mean turning into an automaton who charges through her day without taking time to talk to patients or co-workers. It does meaning avoiding time wasters, and recognizing your most important tasks and doing them first.

Start Early

Rushing in to work just in the nick of time or a few minutes late can mess up your entire day. You're tense and stressed, and co-workers on the previous shift -- who want to go home -- are aggravated. You might miss crucial information because your mind isn't settled into work mode yet. Getting to work a few minutes early helps you start the day calmly.

Organize Your Supplies

"A place for everything and everything in its place" is an essential axiom for nurses. Start with your pockets; don't just throw your phone, alcohol wipes, pens, hand sanitizer, reading glasses, scissors and tape in willy-nilly; use a pocket organizer so you can get to things easily when you need them. After report, take a minute to look at your patient's immediate needs so you can gather supplies you need before heading down the hall. If a patient needs a new IV so you can start her antibiotics, take everything with you so you don't have to backtrack. If you keep supplies in each room, check to make sure everything is stocked in the morning. Restock for the next shift at the end of your day.

Do What's Important First

If you've been a nurse for any length of time, you know you won't get everything done that you'd like to do. Unfortunately, spending time with patients generally takes a hit as you try to get the scheduled meds, treatments, and basic care done. Prioritize your list to make sure you don't miss any essentials. Some nurses rely on a preprinted scheduling chart including each patient and their essential treatments. Check off tasks as you do them so you don't surprise a patient by trying to change her dressing twice in one shift.

Organized nurses use anything from clipboards to smartphone apps –just figure out what works best for you. I always use one standard report sheet when getting and giving report, and color coding will become your best friend!

*You can get access to my favorite ICU friendly and multi-patient report sheets on my website: www.ontargetnurse.com

Organize Your Report

No one wants to be the nurse who gives a report in disjointed segments, pieces of paper spilling over the table and lots of backtracking to mention things she forgot to tell you about a previous patient. A preprinted form can also help you organize your report, with spaces for current meds, treatments and any changes in orders.

Professional Challenges

A nurse's obligations aren't limited to clinical care. One must also adhere to legal and ethical standards in addition to maintaining professional relationships with colleagues. Before any nurse takes an action regarding patient care, they must consider the facility's policies, federal health care laws and what's in the best interest of the patient. As a nurse you must also ensure you act in a way that supports the rest of the team and encourages a high level of patient care.

Nursing is a profession that can be both rewarding and challenging at the same time. Since nurses represent the majority of the workforce, they are often targeted by hospitals as a way to cut down their healthcare costs. Nurses play a very important role in the medical industry. Known for their most caring traits, nurses have now developed their own reputation and identity in the health care area.

But despite being recognized and valued, nurses still have to face several difficulties and challenges in their profession. Some of these challenges are easy to overcome but others are quite complicated for the nurses to handle. Given below are some of the major challenges that nurses are facing today:

Long Working Hours

Hospitals usually have long working hours and re□uire nurses to work in long shifts. But in many cases nurses are assigned shifts in a back-to-back manner, right after the other. The job of a nurse is a tedious one and requires an individual to have great strength of mind along with having a gentle attitude towards the patients.

Being a nurse, you'll face quite a lot of fatigue and feel like you have too many responsibilities with too little time. You will be required to administer medications, assess patients, do paperwork and perform treatments regularly. To carry out all this effectively, you need to plan ahead by organizing your tasks and sorting out your priorities. Create a flexible schedule that will assist you in your most hectic shifts.

Safety

Nurses must vigilantly follow safety procedures to protect themselves, their patients, and other hospital staff. They must also assess the safety and cleanliness of patient environments and monitor the procedures used by the facility and fellow health care staff. If a nurse notices that patient rooms are not being adequately cleaned and disinfected, she has a responsibility to bring it to the attention of hospital management or take action herself. This also applies if she notes that nurses or staff are not following hospital or legal guidelines regarding hand washing, disposal of syringes or other hazards.

Workplace Violence

Another major challenge that nurses face is the violent behavior of patients in the hospital. Many patients are difficult to handle and can be violent at times. This is why this profession is highly demanding and quite stressful at times.

Workplace violence is a serious problem among nurses. Most of the time, patients and co-workers (physicians and other nurses) are the major sources of violence against nurses. If you find any type of violent behavior in the workplace, report it directly to your supervisor, since it is the sole responsibility of the hospital administration to monitor any violent activity in the premises.

Exposure To Diseases

Since nurses are responsible to look after the patients, they are always at the risk of being exposed to various diseases that these patients have. Many times, even the healthiest of the nurses catch these illnesses. It is imperative that the nurse to take care of him or herself by fortifying him/herself with the proper vitamins/nutrition, keeping up to date with his/her vaccinations, and staying physically fit.

There are many studies that report work-related injuries and diseases among nurses. Occupational health nurses play an important role here. Nurses should explore new strategies to help identify the potential seriousness of workplace injuries and illnesses. They should also advocate for better health and safety policies by monitoring the workplace and directly reporting the issues to the hospital management.

Workplace Relationships

Caring for patients requires a team effort, so it's crucial that nurses work well with fellow nurses and with physicians and other health care specialists. If they don't, they may spend more time disagreeing than helping patients recover. In a high-pressure environment such as a medical facility, it's inevitable that tensions will sometimes run high and spark conflict. Repeated conflict can permanently damage working relationships among staff, causing communication breakdowns and hindering the department's ability to provide adequate patient care.

Shortage of Nursing Staff

Hospitals are facing crisis in managing and maintaining adequate nursing staff. This is because hospital CEOs are investing more in advanced medical technologies rather than focusing on maintaining proper staff. Due to the increasing demand for nurses, the nurse to patient ratio remains unbalanced. The number of patients is increasing day by day and there is an acute shortage of nurses to attend the patients.

Conclusion

You have worked hard to get to where you are, and the next step is to land in the right place. With the rush at the end of the semester, the celebrations of graduation, and the pressure to find a job, it feels like you have been catapulted into a new life.

During your first 100 days or sooner, you'll begin to understand the difference between nursing school and the real world. Expect a seemingly endless string of eye-opening experiences. Just keep focused. Remind yourself that for the time that you are on the job, your patients are the most important thing in your life. Your observations, even as a new nurse, can be critical to their recovery.

Then, when your shift is over, leave your work at the office or hospital. Your career may depend on it. Nurse burnout is a serious problem, causing a steadily increasing exodus from the profession. A study done in 2007 by Dr. Christine Cover reported that 13% of new nurses left their primary job, while 37% were planning to leave.[1] At the minimum, those nurses are essentially wasting four years of a costly university education. More importantly, they are closing the door to the many opportunities that nursing can offer. To keep from joining the exodus, be selfish about your free time. Give yourself plenty of opportunity to unwind, particularly after a difficult shift. Find ways to relieve stress when you are away from the job.

Consider the first 100 days as an important transition in your career and your life. The best pathway to success during this time is to go into your job well prepared with information you have gathered during your education and the hiring process. Watch, listen and learn. And realize that this period is an important part of your professional growth.

They may forget your name,

but they will never forget how you made them feel

-Maya Angelou

Other Resources Written by Jay:

- Other 10 Benefits of Joining Professional Nursing Organizations and Associations
- 3 Tips on How to be a Critical Care Nurse for New Grad Nurses
- My NCLEX Experience: Study Tips and Resources for Nursing Students

To Connect With Jay:

Website: www.ontargetnurse.com

Email: jay@ontargetnurse.com

Instagram:@jvogue92

YouTube: www.youtube.com/jayquinn92

1. AACN. (2019). Nursing Shortage. Retrieved from https://www.aacnnursing.org/News-Information/Fact-Sheets/Nursing-Shortage

www.ingramcontent.com/pod-product-compliance
Lightning Source LLC
Chambersburg PA
CBHW071444170526
45158CB00005BA/1833